# Understanding
# Reiki

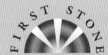

FIRST STONE

# Contents

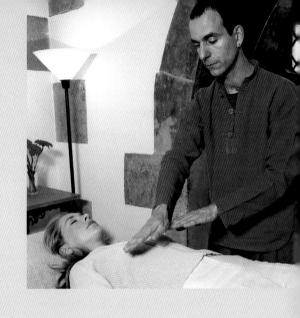

# 1

# Introducing Reiki

**R**eiki is a unique system of energy healing. It is practised by transmitting a spiritually guided 'life force' through the hands.

Since ancient times various methods for healing with subtle energies (also called natural life energies) have been in use.

It was in the early 20th century that a Japanese doctor, Mikao Usui, developed one of the most powerful yet gentle ways of healing with natural life energy.

He used his body as a channel for this subtle energy and transmitted it through his hands to others. Usui

> *He used his body as a channel for natural life energy*

called his method the "Usui Reiki Ryoho", which translates as the Usui System of Natural Healing with Universal Life Energy. Today his method is simply called Reiki.

The ability to perform Reiki is passed on through an initiation process from teacher to student.

Reiki is being practised around the world by an estimated two million practitioners and has become one of the fastest growing complementary therapies of our time.

## WHAT DOES REIKI MEAN?

When we translate the Japanese term 'Reiki' into English, we see the word has two components:

- **Rei** meaning Universal Consciousness, Spirit or the Hidden Source
- **Ki** meaning Life Energy or Life Force.

Put together, Reiki means Spiritual Life Force.

## REI

Rei can be thought of as a universal field of consciousness

that is composed neither of matter nor energy but has the primary organising power to create life from both. Rei is the mind of nature, an infinite intelligence that is able to design and harmonise the vast number of events that life creates at any moment in time.

*To help you understand this concept, imagine nature to be an ocean.*

As you look across the surface of the vast expanse of water, you see waves rising and falling everywhere in perfect rhythm. Rei is the ocean's 'spirit', creating and organising all the waves you can see.

Individual life forms in nature rise from Rei just as the waves rise from the ocean. In the same way that each wave is an expression of the ocean, so each individual life form is an expression of Rei.

As the winds and the tidal forces provide the energy for the waves to rise, it is the force that the Japanese call Ki that provides the energy for living organisms to exist and to thrive.

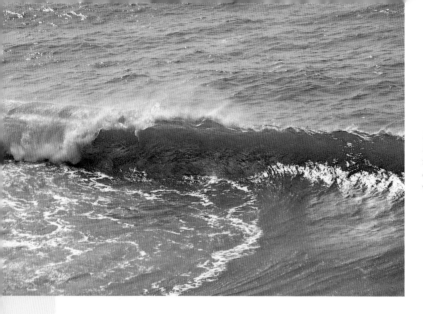

*In deep: Rei is like the spirit of the ocean, organising the waves.*

## KI

Ki, the life energy within all living beings, has many names:

- The Chinese call it 'Chi'
- The Indians named it 'Prana'
- The Sufis call it 'Baraka'.

In recent decades, science has developed instruments that are sensitive enough to detect and measure aspects of Ki. It can be described as a living electromagnetic energy that is being absorbed, stored and distributed by living cells.

Most Eastern healing practices are based on an awareness of Ki. Good health is usually defined as the state where Ki flows through the body in a free and balanced way.

Ill health is the state where the flow of the life energy is continuously impeded by stress and tension so that areas of stagnant energy develop, leading to pain and other symptoms of illness.

Most traditional Eastern healing practices aim at restoring a healthy flow of Ki in the body. Reiki not only does this but goes even further. While the Ki that is currently present in the body is being rebalanced, additional Ki is made available through the practitioner, who acts as a channel for the Life Force.

As a result, the receiver's 'batteries' are recharged more quickly and the healing process can be completed more easily and thoroughly.

## INTELLIGENT ENERGY

Reiki is a conscious and intelligent energy that flows through and nourishes all life. It can only do good, as it is life energy expressed and guided by Spirit (Rei). 'Spirit' or 'spiritual' refers to a hidden source that maintains, interconnects and evolves all life. While every religion has its own ideas and names for this source of life, Rei transcends specific religious beliefs.

Consequently, Reiki is not a religious practice but a way to support natural healing for everyone everywhere, regardless of their background and beliefs.

'Spiritual energy' and 'life

force' may appear to be mysterious terms that we do not fully understand. Yet everyday things such as electrical currents or even the pull of gravity are really just as mysterious.

Electricity is made up of sub-atomic particles called electrons, which flow to create a current. To date, scientists have been unable to explain exactly what an electron is and what creates it.

Does this prevent you from plugging in your kettle? Your cup of tea is the result of an unresolved scientific mystery. Should this keep you from enjoying it? Scientists still do not really know what gravity is, and yet we experience its power every moment of our lives.

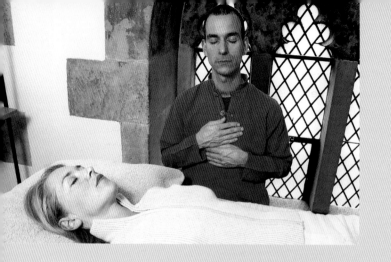

# 2 A Brief History

**T**he Reiki method of natural healing was discovered and developed in the early 20th century by Dr. Mikao Usui.

He was born in 1865 in a small Japanese village near present-day Nagoya. In his early life, Usui studied and practised a Japanese form of energy work called Kiko, which involved meditation, breathing and moving exercises similar to the methods of Tai Chi and Chi Kung.

The practice of Kiko also included techniques for healing through the laying on of hands. The hands-on healing techniques of Kiko required practitioners to first build up their own personal energy through meditation and energising exercises.

Thereafter they were able to pass on some of their energy to another person through the laying on of hands. But this way of working left the practitioner depleted and tired at the end of the treatment.

Usui knew that the world's

13

spiritual traditions were rich in accounts of healers who, for the purpose of helping others to heal, drew on an energy source greater than themselves.

## HEALERS

Sometimes these practitioners were mystics, saints or shamans. Often they were 'normal' people who had discovered their ability to heal by accident.

What they all had in common was the ability to channel healing energies from an inexhaustible source. They allowed the subtle forces of nature to work through them, and felt uplifted and refreshed after giving a treatment.

Usui felt that everyone had the potential to become such a healer. Inspired by this intuition he decided to dedicate his life to finding out how humans can connect with the infinite source (Rei) and help others to heal.

His quest led him on extensive travels through Japan, China, Tibet, Northern India and Europe. In his desire to learn ways in which to connect with nature's inexhaustible energy, Usui studied a wide range of subjects, including psychology, medicine, spiritual and psychic development and the world's religions.

However, the more knowledge Usui accumulated the more he felt like a chef who had built an impressive collection of the world's most sophisticated recipes without yet having found the actual ingredients.

Usui became a leading civil servant, and he was successful as a business man. But after some years, Usui decided to continue his original quest for the infinite source of healing energy by living a life in meditation. He became a Buddhist monk and lived a monk's life for the next seven years.

## RETREAT

One springtime, Usui went on a 21-day retreat to meditate and fast on Mt. Kurama, a sacred mountain situated at the northern end of Kyoto.

15

Towards the end of his retreat, Usui had a profoundly transforming spiritual experience. He described it as a great light entering through the top of his head and attuning his entire being to the Reiki energy.

Immediately thereafter he found his healing abilities to be greatly enhanced – without his own energy being depleted after treating others.

He was filled with joy and gratitude for his new gift and soon went on to initiate others into Reiki and to teach the healing techniques he had developed.

## TRAINING

In April 1922, Usui moved to Tokyo and founded the Usui Reiki Healing Society (Usui Reiki Ryoho Gakkai). A year later, a devastating earthquake hit Japan. Usui and his students offered all the help they could.

Word of the success of Reiki treatment soon spread. Before his death on 9th March 1926, Mikao Usui had taught Reiki to more than 2,000 students and had trained 16 Reiki teachers.

One of the teachers trained by Usui was Dr. Chujiro Hayashi, who started his own Reiki school and clinic in Tokyo.

In 1935 a Japanese woman who lived in Hawaii came to Hayashi's clinic to receive treatment for a gall bladder disease. Her name was Hawayo Takata. After successful treatment, Takata became one of Hayashi's students, and she went on to bring Reiki to the Western world.

After Hayashi had trained Takata as a teacher in 1938, she began to teach Reiki in Hawaii and later on the American mainland.

After Hawayo Takata's death in 1980, the 22 teachers she trained continued to spread the Reiki method of natural healing across the USA, Europe and India. But it was not until the mid-1990s that Western and Japanese Reiki practitioners began to communicate and share developments.

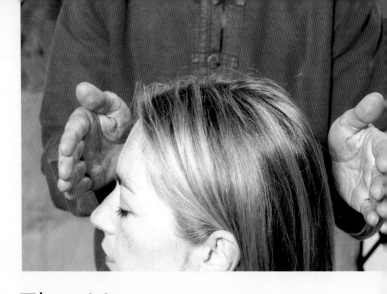

# The Human
# Energy Field

The human body is surrounded by a field of energy often referred to as the aura. Most people can sense it and refer to the 'vibes' or 'feel' of a person.

Some children can see the aura and some keep this ability as adults. Almost everyone can learn to see at least the inner layer of the aura.

When I teach it in my advanced Reiki classes, a typical response from students is: "I've seen this before sometimes, but I've never paid attention to it."

Reality is shaped by what we pay attention to. Long before a symptom develops in the physical body, its 'blueprint' appears as a pattern of disruption in the aura.

SENSING TENSION

These early warning signs can be detected, and people often sense them as states of tension, unrest or discomfort long before any illness occurs.

Today we know that living cell tissue stores and transmits energy. Science is now able to

19

confirm a wide range of energies that sustain the human aura.

These include subtle electrical currents, magnetic and electromagnetic energies and light (so called 'bio-photons'), as well as heat and sound.

## GOING ON-LINE

The aura serves as a kind of bio-energetic Internet, and each one of the several billion cells in the body is constantly 'on-line', receiving and feeding back information.

Without this communication, none of the vital bodily functions (such as metabolism, cell replacement and the immune response) would be possible.

The aura is the organising 'body wide web' that holds things together in a synchronised, harmonious way.

Every human energy field develops its own unique frequency. Human auras interact with each other as well as interacting with the energy fields of animals and plants.

The longer and more intimate the interaction between the individuals, the greater the exchange between their energy fields. Have you ever wondered why couples often look alike after decades of being together, or why dogs frequently develop traits similar to those of their owners?

Every energy field contains an abundance of information and reflects physical, emotional, mental and spiritual aspects of the individual.

The aura is an information network and a highly sensitive perceptual system. It keeps us in constant communication with everything around us.

The power of the Reiki System of Natural Healing lies in the fact that it works directly with the aura.

The aura is in constant movement as energy flows into and out from it. Within this flow and exchange, certain focal points anchor the aura into the physical body.

## THE CHAKRAS
These focal points are called

the 'chakras' – which translates as 'wheels' in Indian Sanskrit.

The chakras are for energy what the mouth is for food and drink, and the nose, for air. Yet they are more than just openings for energy. They mediate all energy within, coming into, and going out of, the body, as well as playing a major part in the distribution of energy for the physical, emotional, mental and spiritual aspects of our being. The chakras also play a major part in the distribution of energy for the physical, emotional, mental and spiritual needs.

There are seven major chakras, lined up from the top of the head down to the base of the spine. The sites of the seven main chakras correspond to the sites of the main glands forming the endocrine system, which regulates all other body functions via the hormones. During a Reiki treatment, the practitioner focuses on the receiver's chakras, as they are the primary access to the human energy system.

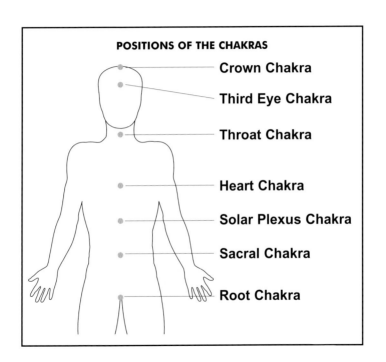

**POSITIONS OF THE CHAKRAS**

Crown Chakra

Third Eye Chakra

Throat Chakra

Heart Chakra

Solar Plexus Chakra

Sacral Chakra

Root Chakra

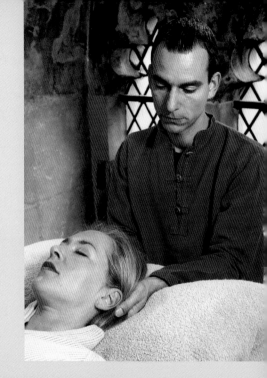

# 4

# How
# Does
# Reiki
# Work?

**R**eiki is a gentle yet powerful way of healing through the human energy field (aura), treating physical, emotional, mental and spiritual imbalances.

Reiki is conscious life energy and is able to detect and reach the root cause of a condition.

For example, if the root cause of a migraine is chronic dehydration, Reiki helps increase the instinctive desire to drink more water.

If the root cause of a stomach ulcer is bottled-up anger, Reiki aids its release and restores emotional balance. Our bodies have an in-built tendency to maintain good health.

Reiki supports nature in doing its job. The question is not so much how we can be healed, but how we managed to get ill against nature's intention in the first place.

Stop for a moment and imagine that you are looking at your life as an 'energy investment banker'. Pay attention to how you currently invest your life energy:

- Are you doing the work you love and do you love the

work you do?

- Are you taking good care of your body?
- Are your relationships with others mutually fulfilling?
- Do you feel that your life is going somewhere meaningful?
- Do you like and accept yourself?
- Have you chosen a supportive environment?
- Do you focus on the positive things in your life?

If you've answered every question with 'yes' – congratulations! If you've answered some of the questions with 'no', then it is likely that conflicts, resistance and stagnation are consuming some of your life energy.

It takes more energy to stop yourself from being, doing and having what you want than it takes to achieve it! This is where Reiki can unfold its greatest power for you. Reiki rekindles a thirst for life. After all it is universal LIFE energy!

It re-ignites the flame, and provides you with the energy to plan meaningful action and carry it through harmoniously.

Reiki stories from around the world can fill volumes with accounts of positive transformations. A few examples with my own clients and students: the ability to quit smoking easily, to heal issues or conditions that had been part of their lives for years, to make positive changes in their careers, feeling a deep sense of connectedness with all life, experiencing heightened intuition, emotional balance and a general sense of increased personal energy.

Reiki is channelled by the practitioner, and transmitted to the receiver primarily through the hands. It is not the practitioner's own personal energy that is being used. The practitioner is given the ability to channel the Universal Life Energy during training.

NATURAL LIFE ENERGY
Reiki is a natural expression of life's infinite intelligence and can only do good.

No conscious effort in allowing the energy to work is required. Reiki communicates intelligently with the receiver's body-mind and goes to where it's needed. This works just as the oxygen we inhale, and the nutrients we consume don't need to be guided by our conscious mind to the part of the body that needs them.

## SELF-HEALING

Healing is ultimately a journey towards wholeness. The words 'heal', 'whole' and 'holy' share the same source in language. Intention, the desire for well-being, is the driving force on this journey. A Reiki practitioner helps to make more life energy available to the receiver so that the body-mind can fully activate its self-healing powers.

The receiver's body-mind is responsible for the effects it creates from 'miraculous' healing to no noticeable effects at the time.

A Reiki treatment is non-intrusive and non-manipulative. It invites the receiver to draw the energy they need through (not from) the practitioner. No abuse of Reiki is possible because its inherent intent is to heal and make whole.

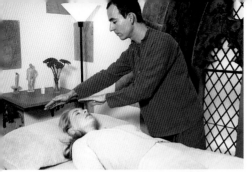

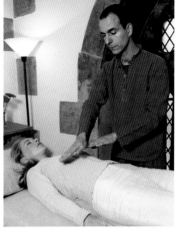

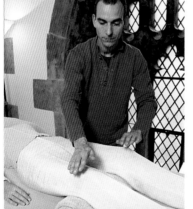

## AURA CLEANSING/SWEEPING

*Clockwise from top left – demonstrating the process of aura cleansing and sweeping. The Reiki practitioner moves the hands in a sweeping movement from the client's head downwards.*

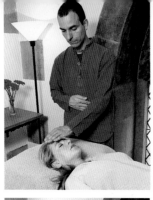

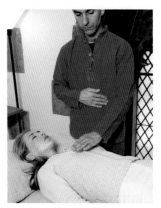

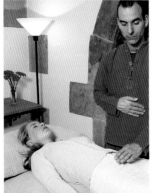

## SCANNING THE ENERGY

*Clockwise from top left – the practitioner uses his hand to tune in to individual chakras so he can sense their state.*

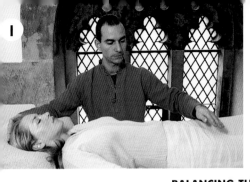
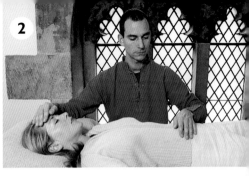

## BALANCING THE CHAKRAS

**1**. *Balancing the Root Chakra with the Crown Chakra.* **2**. *Balancing the Sacral Chakra with the Third Eye Chakra.* **3**. *Balancing the Solar Plexus with the Throat Chakra.* **4**. *Treating the Heart Chakra on its own.*

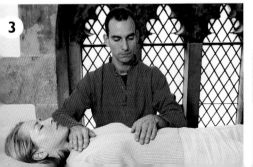
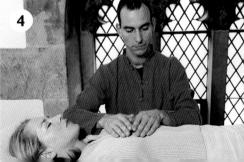

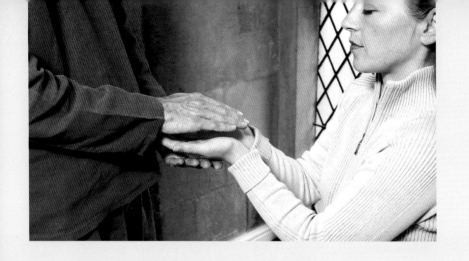

# 5 The Main Benefits Of Reiki

**R**eiki is a method for supporting the body and mind's natural self-healing abilities in ways that are non-intrusive and non-manipulative, so everyone can benefit from it at any age.

There are almost no limits to the use of Reiki. It is compatible with other forms of treatment and has no negative side effects.

You don't have to believe in Reiki in order to benefit from it. No faith or conviction is required other than the belief that it is possible for you to be healed and that you deserve to get better.

As Reiki is a complementary treatment, it should never be used as a replacement for any medical treatment. If a person needs diagnosis and medical treatment, they should see a medical doctor.

A Reiki treatment does not 'cure' medical conditions – it simply assists people in becoming healthier. However, Reiki can offer much help when other approaches have exhausted their possibilities.

## TREATMENTS

The number of treatments required varies from case to case. Generally speaking, any number between three and ten one-hour sessions will bring significant benefits.

The interval between treatments may vary. Sometimes daily treatment may be required, at other times weekly to monthly treatments will suffice.

Animals and plants are sentient beings too, and can benefit from Reiki.

The distance healing technique even allows the practitioner to help animals when other forms of treatment prove too frightening or uncomfortable.

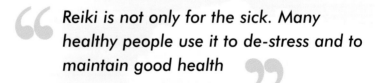

*Reiki is not only for the sick. Many healthy people use it to de-stress and to maintain good health*

## COMMON BENEFITS

- Stress relief. Many diseases result from prolonged stress.
- Deep relaxation.
- Improved sleep.
- Pain relief.
- Detoxification.
- Strengthening of the natural self-healing powers and the immune system.
- An increase in personal energy, vitality and confidence.
- A healthy mind-body connection.
- Comforting feelings of connectedness with all life.
- Release of emotional and energetic blockages.
- Support of one's personal and spiritual growth.
- Balance and inner peace.
- Rejuvenation. Many people look years younger after a Reiki session.

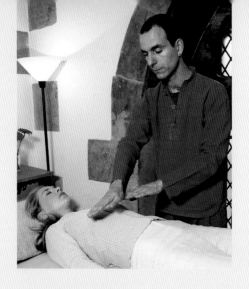

# 6 A Reiki Treatment

**A** **Reiki treatment aims to restore good health and wholeness.**

The healing promoted by Reiki is not medical warfare, where symptoms are being 'fought', stress is 'beaten', pain is 'killed', where we 'wrestle' with an illness and 'battles' are lost or won.

Our language when dealing with illness is littered with violent images in situations where inner peace, integration and forgiveness are needed most urgently.

To understand Reiki, it is important to contrast its methods with other approaches.

Regardless of the techniques or rituals that are employed, any treatments, both conventional and alternative, will always express a certain relationship between the people involved.

This relationship will be guided by attitudes and intentions.

I would like to illustrate this idea by contrasting two different attitudes towards health care.

37

## A CURE – TREATING THE SYMPTOM

During a cure the patient remains fairly passive, waits, hopes, and is seen as a victim of an illness.

The practitioner makes a diagnosis, expects submission from the patient, and prescribes. Such a relationship creates rituals of control and authority.

The practitioner takes the responsibility away from the patient, and much technology is used in the attempt to collect objective data for accurate diagnosis. A highly specialised view determines the practitioner's judgement and choice of action.

The administered treatments aim to remove the symptoms, the physical manifestations of the disease.

The cure is successful when the patient survives the treatments and the symptoms do not.

## A HEALING – TREATING THE ROOT CAUSE

The practitioner attends to the entire person, not just to one organ or one body function.

During the treatment, time is given to discussing and understanding relevant problems, which may be affecting the client's health.

The client is invited to participate in their healing by paying more attention to their needs and trusting their inner intuitive guidance.

The practitioner serves the client as a source of energy, encouragement and guidance, and helps them to become empowered to self-heal more easily.

The treatments aim at recreating balance in a non-invasive way. The healing is successful when the client's energy and well-being have been restored.

When teaching the Usui Reiki Method of Natural Healing, I encourage the students to adopt this attitude towards healing.

## WHAT HAPPENS DURING A REIKI TREATMENT?

A Reiki session is a treat for everyone. During the treatment, you remain dressed, and sit or lie comfortably with cushions, while the practitioner transmits the life energy to you.

Most parts of a Reiki treatment are performed as a series of hand positions, with the practitioner applying his or her hands either with or without touch.

The Reiki energy can be powerfully transmitted while the practitioner holds his or her hands from 1 to 5 inches (2.5 to 12.5 cm) above the client's body, within the energy field (aura).

Many practitioners will include advanced techniques such as aura cleansing, energy scanning and chakra balancing to increase the benefits of the treatment.

Reiki is one of the most comfortable routes to well-being. It can only really be understood when you experience the beauty of this comforting, soothing and strengthening energy flow.

WHAT DOES REIKI FEEL LIKE?
Sometimes, the Reiki energy may give you the feeling that

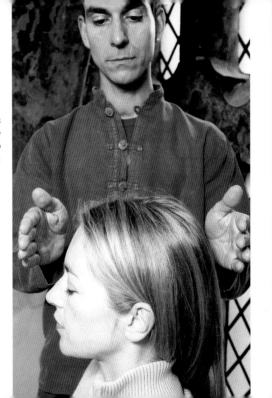

*No touching: Treatment is possible without the practitioner needing to touch the client's body.*

41

you are bathed in light and warmth that reaches deep in to your body and mind. Sometimes, the gentle currents of energy flowing through you may feel like the cleansing water of a refreshing brook.

At other times, Reiki may feel like a spiritual force that dissolves blockages with its subtle vibrations.

The Usui Reiki Method of Natural Healing is gentle and safe, and the benefits of a treatment can stay with you for a long time.

## TREATMENT SET-UP AND STRUCTURE

The Reiki practitioner creates a quiet, comfortable and soothing environment in a room with soft, relaxing music and a pleasant aroma, perhaps from a candle, incense or essential oils.

The receiver should wear comfortable clothes and take off their shoes, watch, glasses and any jewellery.

During the initial interview, the receiver has the opportunity to tell the practitioner why they are

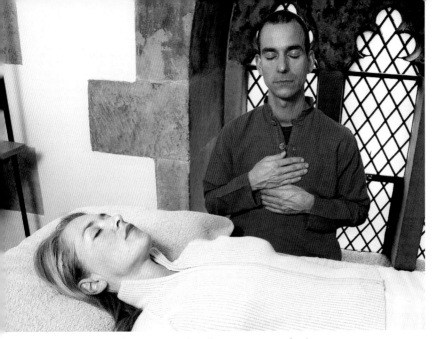

*Calm start: A few moments of meditation to prepare for the treatment.*

43

seeking treatment and how they want Reiki to help.

For the treatment the receiver can sit in a chair or lie down on a mattress, a futon or a treatment couch. Pillows are used to support the head and knees, and sometimes receivers like to be covered with a light blanket.

The practitioner may begin the treatment by preparing him or herself mentally with a few moments of meditation and centring to help them consciously connect with Reiki.

Then they touch the receiver lightly or hold their hands a few inches above the body, staying in each position for three to five minutes. The choice of hand positions and the time spent in each one will depend upon the receiver's needs.

Most of the time, the practitioner will include hand positions that correspond to the major chakras or energy centres in the aura and the body. If there is enough time, both the front and the back of the body will be treated.

## RELAXATION

During the treatment, no conscious effort is required from the receiver. He or she just 'be', noticing what he or she notices. If the mind wanders off, that's fine. Often, the mind relaxes as the body relaxes, and a sense of carefreeness develops as stress and worries dissolve.

The practitioner will usually end a treatment working on the receiver's feet, which ensures an easy return to the waking state. Sufficient time is allowed for the receiver to get up and stretch, and talk about his or her experience of the session.

When you go to see a Reiki practitioner, allow 10-15 minutes of quiet time after the treatment without having to rush somewhere.

The length of an individual Reiki session can be adjusted to the receiver's needs and schedule, with the minimum being 15 minutes and the maximum being around two hours.

# HAND POSITIONS FOR TREATING THE FRONT OF THE BODY – PART 1

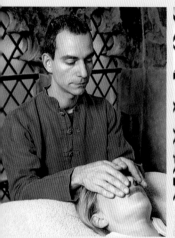

*Treating the eyes and cheeks, Third Eye Chakra.*

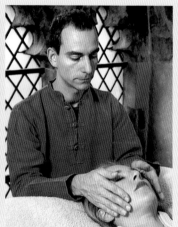

*Treating the temples and jaw.*

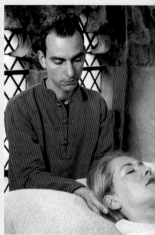

*Treating the back of the head, Third Eye and Crown Chakra.*

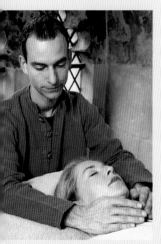

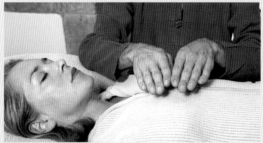

*Above: Treating the upper chest, Heart Chakra.*

*Below: Treating the lower chest, Solar Plexus Chakra.*

*Treating the throat area, Throat Chakra.*

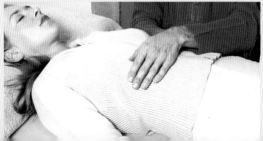

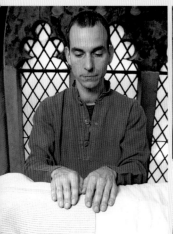

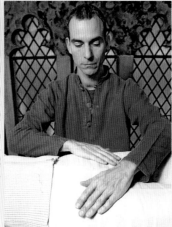

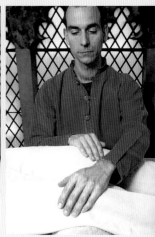

*Treating the abdomen, Sacral Chakra.*

*Treating the lower abdomen, pubic bone, Root Chakra.*

*Treating the knees.*

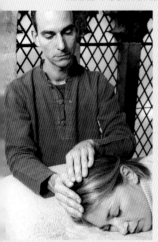

*Treating the crown, Crown Chakra.*

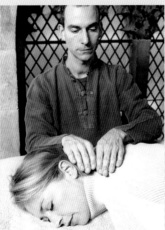

*Treating the neck and upper shoulders, Throat Chakra.*

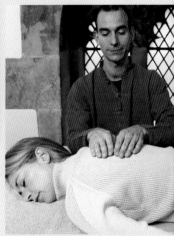

*Treating the shoulder blades, Heart Chakra.*

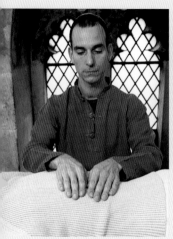

*Treating the lower lungs and kidneys, Solar Plexus Chakra.*

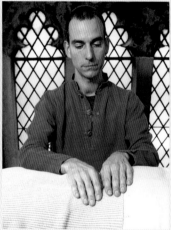

*Treating the lower back, sacrum, Sacral Chakra.*

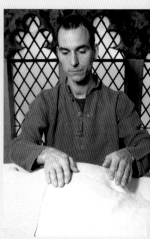

*Treating the coccyx, Root Chakra.*

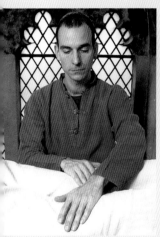

*Treating the back of the knees.*

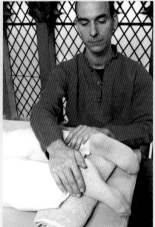

*Treating the ankles.*

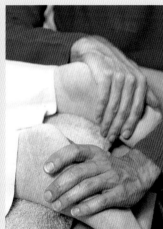

*Treating the feet.*

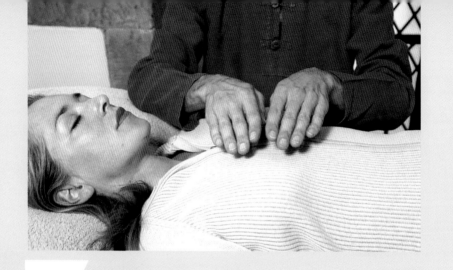

# 7 Case Histories

**H**ealing can imply much more than getting rid of symptoms. It can be a unique journey to wholeness.

Wholeness means that we pay attention to all aspects of our being and integrate them with our daily life.

Reiki is a tremendous support on this journey, giving us both strength and guidance.

I would like to include a few case histories to provide real-life examples of how Reiki affected some of my students and clients.

DAVID

David came to see me because he had been suffering for years from sinusitis. He had lost his sense of smell and frequently suffered from headaches and low energy.

The initial energy scan revealed that not only were his sinuses depleted of energy, but so too were his stomach and intestines. After treating the face for 15 minutes, the headache went but the pain and blockage in the sinuses persisted. I went on to treat key areas of his respiratory

53

system and thereafter his stomach. After five minutes of treating David's stomach, his sinuses began to clear, and after 10 more minutes working on the abdomen, his pain had gone and he was able to breathe freely through his nose for the first time in years.

## MARY

When I first saw Mary, she was going through the break-up of her six-year marriage and desperately needed to relax and collect herself. Her general health was fine, but with the strain of the separation she was experiencing panic attacks at night and was getting very little sleep. She decided to have weekly Reiki treatments.

After her second session, the panic attacks stopped and Mary enjoyed good sleep again. She was very pleased, felt much more balanced, and her natural enthusiasm had returned.

Unfortunately, a few weeks later, Mary had a car crash, which left her with whiplash pain. Her doctor had prescribed painkillers, but Mary found them too strong. She was in agony when I saw her, and I concentrated treatment on her neck, shoulders and entire spine. During her second session following the accident, she gradually felt her pain fade away and left the clinic with full mobility restored.

## RITA

Rita was in distress because of a recent miscarriage. She woke up in the middle of every night and then had difficulty getting back to sleep. During her Reiki treatment, she experienced a pain in her womb that she described as being 'dark and heavy'.

While I treated her abdomen with the laying on of hands, I asked Rita to imagine that the dark heaviness would dissolve and become light. The pain had gone by the end of the session and although Rita was a little dizzy, she felt relieved. When I saw her a week later, she looked much more refreshed and was able to sleep through the night.

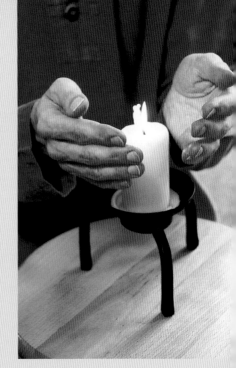

# 8 The Reiki Tradition

**T**he Reiki tradition is not just a system of passing on knowledge and techniques.

There is a unique initiation process, designed to re-ignite the Universal Life Force in the student. Over the years, the Reiki lineage has branched out, with Mikao Usui being the common root. If a teacher's lineage does not go back to Usui, then what they teach is not Reiki.

Reiki is usually taught in three levels or degrees, allowing the student to develop confidence at each level. At the heart of the initiation into each level is a process called the attunement. The attunement is an energy transmission through the teacher to the student.

During this energy transmission, the student's entire being gets in tune with the energy frequency of Reiki. The result is the ability to channel Reiki for him/herself and others for the rest of his or her life.

While the Reiki teacher performs the attunement

process, it is the Universal Life Energy that creates the new practitioner.

The experience of being attuned is different for everyone. Some may feel the energy as heat, or as subtle currents tingling through their bodies; others may see colours, while some may notice hardly anything at first.

Whatever the experience during an attunement may be, it is important not to judge its power and value thereby. The value of an attunement lies in allowing you to perform Reiki and in helping you to improve your life.

## THE THREE LEVELS OF INITIATION

### *REIKI LEVEL ONE*

During the Level One class, the teacher will attune the student to Reiki in a way that enables him or her to use it for self-healing and to pass it on to others simply through the laying on of hands.

The student will learn a series of hand positions, the structure of a healing session, and techniques for aura cleansing and chakra balancing.

They will hear the story of Dr. Usui's quest for this powerful gift and begin to use it during the hands-on practice session. After taking a Level One class, the student is advised to practise on himself or herself as well as on friends and family. This gives the student the time to build confidence and competence with his or her new skills before taking Level Two. Students are usually advised to consider working with the general public only after they have completed the Level Two course.

*REIKI LEVEL TWO*
The highlights of a Level Two class include a further attunement and the initiation into the three sacred Reiki Level Two symbols. These sacred symbols will allow the student to perform distance healing across space and time, and they will learn and practise the relevant applications.

The teacher may choose to provide scientific explanations

for these new skills in energy work. Finally, it is at Level Two when professional practice becomes an important item to be covered.

## REIKI LEVEL THREE

After completing the Reiki Level Two training, the student can take the opportunity to become a teacher in the Usui Reiki Method of Natural Healing.

Level Three will significantly increase the student's personal energy, as well as enabling him or her to assist others in rediscovering and developing the gift of Reiki.

A Level Three training course will include full instruction on how to give the Reiki attunements for all three levels, and how to teach the classes.

There will be an initiation into at least one additional sacred symbol. Most Level Three courses will also cover advanced Reiki techniques, such as setting up Reiki energy grids, interventions for moving stuck energy, and programming crystals with Reiki.

# Finding a Practitioner

Since Reiki has become one of the fastest growing complementary therapies of our time, it is usually easy to find a practitioner in your area.

Go into your local health food shop or public library, where you will often find leaflets on display.

The best method of finding a Reiki practitioner is to call or visit the complementary health clinics in your area. These clinics require a practitioner to be fully qualified, professionally experienced, and insured, so you can be assured of receiving good-quality treatment.

# About the author

Michael Kaufmann lives and
works in London. He is a Reiki
Master, a practitioner of
hypnotherapy and is also a
master practitioner of
neuro-linguistic programming.
He has been teaching all levels
of Reiki since 1997.

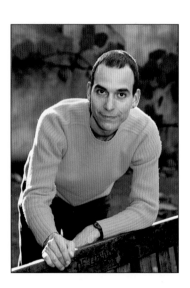

   You can contact him via e-mail
reiki.healing@btopenworld.com
or visit his website:
www.nlp-reiki.co.uk
   Michael teaches monthly Reiki
training courses at The Wren Clinic,
London EC3, tel. 020 7283 8908.